KIDNEY DISEASE DIET BOOK

Heart and Kidney Disease Nutrition Diet Recipes Cookbook

PEYTON AUDREY

ABOUT THE AUTHOR

Peyton Audrey, Registered Dietitian

Peyton Audrey is a highly experienced and dedicated registered dietitian with a profound expertise in the field of nutrition, specifically focused on kidney health. With over 8 years of invaluable experience, Peyton has become a trusted source of guidance and support for individuals seeking to enhance their well-being through dietary choices.

Peyton's passion for nutrition and her commitment to improving the lives of others have been the driving forces behind her successful career. Her knowledge and skills in the realm of kidney health have made her an indispensable resource for those navigating the challenges of managing kidney-related conditions.

Throughout her career, Peyton has worked tirelessly to empower her clients with the knowledge and tools needed to make informed dietary decisions. She understands the unique and nuanced needs of individuals facing kidney health concerns and is dedicated to providing personalized, practical, and effective solutions.

Peyton's commitment to her work extends beyond her professional life; it's a reflection of her genuine desire to make a positive impact on the lives of those she serves. Her approachable and compassionate demeanor, combined with her deep expertise, has earned her the trust and admiration of her clients.

As a registered dietitian, Peyton Audrey strives to create a healthier, more fulfilling future for her clients by helping them harness the power of nutrition. She is committed to making a lasting difference in the lives of those she serves, one meal at a time.

TABLE OF CONTENT

INTRODUCTION: UNDERSTANDING HEART AND KIDNEY DISEASE

HEART AND KIDNEY HEALTH

Heart and kidney health are crucial components of overall well-being, as these two vital organs play essential roles in maintaining the body's proper functioning. Here's an introduction to heart and kidney health:

Heart Health:

1. **Function of the Heart:** The heart is a muscular organ that acts as the body's pump, circulating blood throughout the entire body. It consists of four chambers: two atria and two ventricles. The right side of the heart pumps blood to the lungs for oxygenation, while the left side pumps oxygenated blood to the rest of the body.

2. **Cardiovascular System:** The heart is part of the cardiovascular system, which includes blood vessels like arteries, veins, and capillaries. This system is responsible for delivering oxygen and nutrients to cells, as well as removing waste products.

3. **Factors Affecting Heart Health:** Maintaining a healthy heart involves factors such as a balanced diet, regular exercise, avoiding smoking, limiting alcohol consumption, and managing stress. High blood pressure, high cholesterol levels, and diabetes can also impact heart health.

4. **Heart Diseases:** Heart diseases, such as coronary artery disease, heart failure, and arrhythmias, are

common health issues related to the heart. They can result from atherosclerosis, which is the buildup of plaque in the arteries, or other factors like genetics and lifestyle choices.

5. **Prevention and Treatment:** Preventive measures for heart health include a heart-healthy diet, regular exercise, regular check-ups, and medications if necessary. In severe cases, surgical procedures like bypass surgery or angioplasty may be required.

Kidney Health:

1. **Function of the Kidneys:** The kidneys are bean-shaped organs located on each side of the spine. Their primary function is to filter and remove waste and excess fluid from the bloodstream, which results in the formation of urine. They also help regulate electrolytes, blood pressure, and red blood cell production.

2. **Renal System:** The kidneys are part of the renal system, which also includes the ureters, bladder, and urethra. Together, these organs work to maintain the body's fluid and electrolyte balance.

3. **Factors Affecting Kidney Health:** Kidney health is influenced by factors such as high blood pressure, diabetes, certain medications, and a family history of kidney disease. A balanced diet and adequate hydration are important for preventing kidney issues.

4. **Kidney Diseases:** Kidney diseases can range from mild to severe and can result from various causes, including chronic kidney disease, kidney stones, infections, and autoimmune conditions. Chronic

kidney disease is a progressive condition that can lead to kidney failure if left untreated.

5. **Prevention and Treatment:** Protecting kidney health involves managing underlying conditions like diabetes and hypertension, staying hydrated, and avoiding excessive use of non-prescription pain relievers. In cases of kidney disease, treatment options may include medication, dietary changes, dialysis, or kidney transplantation.

Both heart and kidney health are intertwined with overall well-being, and maintaining these vital organs in good condition is essential for a long and healthy life. Regular medical check-ups and a healthy lifestyle are key to preventing and managing potential issues related to the heart and kidneys.

COMMON CAUSES AND SYMPTOMS

Common causes and symptoms of heart and kidney issues vary depending on the specific condition. Here are some general causes and symptoms for each:

Common Causes and Symptoms of Heart Issues:

1. **Coronary Artery Disease (CAD):**

   - ***Causes:*** Atherosclerosis (buildup of plaque in the arteries), high cholesterol, high blood pressure, smoking, and diabetes.

   - ***Symptoms:*** Chest pain (angina), shortness of breath, fatigue, and in severe cases, heart attack.

2. **Heart Failure:**

   - ***Causes:*** Coronary artery disease, high blood pressure, heart valve disease, and cardiomyopathy.

   - ***Symptoms:*** Fatigue, shortness of breath, swelling in the legs and ankles, rapid or irregular heartbeat.

3. **Arrhythmias:**

   - ***Causes:*** Abnormal electrical activity in the heart, heart attacks, high blood pressure, heart diseases.

   - ***Symptoms:*** Palpitations, dizziness, lightheadedness, chest pain, and fainting.

4. **Valvular Heart Disease:**

- ***Causes***: Congenital heart defects, age-related changes, infection, or damage to heart valves.
- ***Symptoms***: Chest pain, fatigue, shortness of breath, swelling in the feet and ankles.

5. **Hypertension (High Blood Pressure):**

   - ***Causes:*** Genetics, poor diet, lack of exercise, smoking, excessive alcohol consumption, and stress.
   - ***Symptoms:*** Often, high blood pressure has no noticeable symptoms, but it can lead to serious complications over time.

Common Causes and Symptoms of Kidney Issues:

1. **Chronic Kidney Disease (CKD):**

   - ***Causes:*** Diabetes, high blood pressure, glomerulonephritis, polycystic kidney disease, and urinary tract obstructions.
   - ***Symptoms:*** Fatigue, swelling in the hands and feet, changes in urine output, blood in urine, and high blood pressure.

2. **Kidney Stones:**

   - ***Causes:*** Dehydration, high levels of certain minerals in the urine, family history, and dietary factors.
   - ***Symptoms:*** Intense pain in the back or side, blood in urine, frequent urination, and nausea.

3. **Urinary Tract Infections (UTIs):**

   - ***Causes:*** Bacterial infection in the urinary tract.

   - ***Symptoms:*** Frequent urination, burning sensation during urination, cloudy or bloody urine, and abdominal pain.

4. **Acute Kidney Injury (AKI):**

   - ***Causes:*** Sudden and severe loss of kidney function, often due to infections, dehydration, medications, or trauma.

   - ***Symptoms:*** Decreased urine output, swelling, confusion, nausea, and fatigue.

5. **Polycystic Kidney Disease (PKD):**

   - ***Causes:*** Genetic mutation.

   - ***Symptoms:*** Abdominal pain, high blood pressure, and kidney cysts that can lead to kidney failure.

It's important to note that many heart and kidney issues may progress with mild or no symptoms in the early stages. Regular check-ups with a healthcare provider can help detect and manage these conditions early, potentially preventing further complications. If you experience any concerning symptoms related to your heart or kidneys, seeking medical attention promptly is essential.

IMPORTANCE OF NUTRITION IN DISEASE MANAGEMENT

Nutrition plays a crucial role in disease management across a wide range of health conditions. Proper nutrition can have a significant impact on preventing, controlling, and improving the outcomes of various diseases. Here's an overview of the importance of nutrition in disease management:

1. **Prevention of Chronic Diseases:** A healthy and balanced diet can help prevent chronic diseases such as heart disease, diabetes, obesity, and certain types of cancer. For example, reducing the intake of saturated fats, salt, and added sugars while increasing the consumption of fruits, vegetables, whole grains, and lean proteins can lower the risk of these conditions.

2. **Control of Chronic Diseases:** Nutrition is a cornerstone in the management of chronic diseases. For individuals already living with conditions like diabetes, hypertension, or heart disease, a well-planned diet can help manage these conditions effectively. Proper nutrition can help control blood sugar levels, reduce blood pressure, and manage cholesterol levels.

3. **Weight Management:** Maintaining a healthy weight is essential in the management of various health conditions. Nutrition plays a fundamental role in achieving and sustaining a healthy weight. A balanced diet, along with appropriate portion

control, can help individuals reach their weight management goals.

4. **Optimizing Medication Effectiveness:** For individuals taking medications for various conditions, proper nutrition can impact the effectiveness of these drugs. Some medications may require specific dietary considerations, and certain nutrients can interact with medications. A healthcare provider can provide guidance on how to optimize medication effectiveness through diet.

5. **Gastrointestinal Disorders:** Nutrition is particularly crucial in managing gastrointestinal disorders such as irritable bowel syndrome (IBS), celiac disease, and Crohn's disease. Dietary modifications, such as avoiding trigger foods or adhering to a gluten-free diet, can alleviate symptoms and improve quality of life.

6. **Nutrient Deficiencies:** Certain diseases or conditions may lead to nutrient deficiencies. For instance, individuals with malabsorption disorders, like celiac disease or inflammatory bowel disease, may require special diets or supplements to compensate for nutrient losses.

7. **Cancer Management:** Proper nutrition can help cancer patients manage symptoms, improve their nutritional status, and support the body's ability to tolerate cancer treatments like chemotherapy and radiation. A registered dietitian can provide tailored nutrition recommendations for cancer patients.

8. **Autoimmune Disorders:** Nutrition can play a role in managing autoimmune disorders by reducing inflammation and managing symptoms. Anti-inflammatory diets, such as the Mediterranean diet, may be beneficial for individuals with conditions like rheumatoid arthritis and lupus.

9. **Neurological Disorders:** Nutritional strategies, including specific diets like the ketogenic diet for epilepsy or the Mediterranean diet for Alzheimer's disease, can be employed in the management of various neurological conditions.

10. **Mental Health:** Emerging research suggests that nutrition can influence mental health conditions such as depression and anxiety. A balanced diet with adequate nutrients, such as omega-3 fatty acids and B vitamins, may have a positive impact on mental well-being.

In summary, nutrition is a fundamental component of disease management. It can prevent the onset of many chronic conditions, assist in controlling those conditions when they do occur, and improve the overall quality of life for individuals dealing with various health issues. Patients should work closely with healthcare providers and registered dietitians to develop personalized nutrition plans tailored to their specific health needs.

CHAPTER ONE

NUTRITIONAL BASICS

Key Nutrients for Heart and Kidney Health

Maintaining heart and kidney health requires a balanced diet that includes specific nutrients known to support these organs. Here are key nutrients for heart and kidney health:

Key Nutrients for Heart Health:

1. **Omega-3 Fatty Acids:** These essential fatty acids, found in fatty fish (like salmon, mackerel, and sardines), flaxseeds, and walnuts, can help reduce inflammation, lower triglycerides, and improve heart health. Omega-3s may also reduce the risk of irregular heartbeats and lower blood pressure.

2. **Fiber:** Dietary fiber from sources like whole grains, fruits, vegetables, and legumes helps lower cholesterol levels and manage blood pressure. It also promotes weight management and helps regulate blood sugar levels.

3. **Antioxidants (Vitamins C and E, and Beta-Carotene):** Antioxidant-rich foods like fruits and vegetables can protect your heart by reducing oxidative stress and inflammation. Citrus fruits, berries, nuts, and seeds are good sources of these nutrients.

4. **Potassium:** Adequate potassium intake, primarily from foods like bananas, oranges, potatoes, and

spinach, can help lower blood pressure and reduce the risk of heart disease.

5. **Magnesium:** Magnesium, found in foods like nuts, seeds, whole grains, and leafy green vegetables, plays a role in maintaining normal heart rhythm and supporting cardiovascular health.

6. **Calcium:** While calcium is important for bone health, it's also necessary for muscle and nerve function, including the heart. Dairy products, fortified plant-based milks, and leafy greens are good sources of calcium.

7. **Coenzyme Q10 (CoQ10):** CoQ10 is involved in energy production in cells, including heart cells. It may help improve heart function and reduce the side effects of certain heart medications. CoQ10 supplements are available, but it's also present in foods like organ meats, fish, and whole grains.

8. **Garlic:** Garlic has been linked to heart health benefits, including reducing cholesterol levels and blood pressure. It can be consumed in various dishes or as a dietary supplement.

Key Nutrients for Kidney Health:

1. **Potassium:** Adequate potassium intake is essential for maintaining proper kidney function. However, in cases of kidney disease, excessive potassium intake can be harmful. A healthcare provider or registered dietitian can offer guidance on potassium intake for individuals with kidney issues.

2. **Phosphorus:** In kidney disease, phosphorus levels can become imbalanced, and too much phosphorus in the blood can harm the bones and cardiovascular system. Limiting high-phosphorus foods like processed meats, dairy products, and some carbonated beverages may be necessary.

3. **Protein:** Adequate protein intake is important for overall health, but in advanced kidney disease, protein intake may need to be moderated to reduce the workload on the kidneys. This should be done under the guidance of a healthcare provider.

4. **Sodium:** High sodium intake can contribute to high blood pressure, which is a risk factor for kidney disease. Reducing sodium in the diet by avoiding processed and salty foods can help protect kidney health.

5. **Fluids:** Proper fluid management is vital for individuals with kidney issues, especially those on dialysis. Monitoring fluid intake to avoid excessive fluid retention is crucial.

6. **Vitamin D:** Adequate vitamin D is important for kidney health as it helps regulate calcium and phosphorus levels. In some cases of kidney disease, vitamin D supplements may be necessary.

Individual dietary recommendations for heart and kidney health may vary depending on an individual's specific health status and medical conditions. It is important to work with a healthcare provider or registered dietitian to develop a personalized nutrition plan that considers your specific needs and goals.

Reading food labels and practicing portion control are essential skills for making informed and healthy dietary choices. These practices can help you manage your calorie intake, monitor nutrient content, and maintain a balanced diet. Here's how to read food labels and practice portion control effectively:

Reading Food Labels:

1. **Serving Size:** Start by looking at the serving size listed on the label. This information is crucial because all the other values (calories, nutrients) are based on this serving size. Make sure to compare it to the amount you plan to consume.

2. **Calories:** Check the number of calories per serving. This is an important indicator of the energy content of the food. Be mindful of how many servings you plan to eat, as this affects your overall calorie intake.

3. **Nutrient Content:** Examine the amounts of key nutrients such as fat, saturated fat, trans fat, cholesterol, sodium, carbohydrates, fiber, sugars, and protein. Pay attention to the percentages (% Daily Value) provided, which indicate how much a single serving contributes to your daily nutrient needs based on a 2,000-calorie diet. Aim to limit saturated fats, trans fats, cholesterol, and sodium, while prioritizing fiber and essential vitamins and minerals.

4. **Ingredients List:** Review the ingredients list to understand what's in the product. Ingredients are listed in descending order by weight, with the primary ingredient listed first. Be cautious of foods with long lists of unfamiliar or highly processed ingredients.

5. **Nutrition Claims:** Be aware of nutrition claims such as "low-fat," "high-fiber," or "sugar-free." These can provide a quick reference but may not always tell the whole story. It's still important to read the nutrition label for the complete picture.

6. **Allergen Information:** Check for allergen information if you have food allergies or sensitivities. Labels typically highlight common allergens like peanuts, tree nuts, dairy, soy, wheat, and shellfish.

Practicing Portion Control:

1. **Use Measuring Tools:** To understand what a proper portion size looks like, use measuring cups, kitchen scales, and other tools to quantify your food. This can help you visualize appropriate portions.

2. **Learn Visual Cues:** Over time, you can develop an eye for estimating portion sizes without measuring tools. For example, a serving of meat or fish should be about the size of a deck of cards, and a half-cup of pasta is approximately the size of a hockey puck.

3. **Use Smaller Plates:** Eating from smaller plates can help trick your mind into feeling satisfied with smaller portions. Avoid using oversized dinnerware.

4. **Don't Eat Directly from Packaging:** When eating snacks or packaged foods, pour a reasonable portion into a bowl or plate rather than eating directly from the bag or container. It's easier to overindulge when you don't see how much you're consuming.

5. **Listen to Your Body:** Pay attention to hunger and fullness cues. Eat slowly, savor your food, and stop when you feel comfortably full, even if there's food left on your plate.

6. **Plan and Pre-portion:** Pre-plan your meals and snacks, and portion them into containers ahead of time. This prevents mindless overeating and promotes portion control.

By incorporating these practices into your daily routine, you can make healthier choices, control your calorie intake, and better manage your nutrient consumption. This can contribute to a balanced and nutritious diet, which is essential for overall health and well-being.

DIETARY RESTRICTIONS AND CONSIDERATIONS

Dietary restrictions and considerations can be necessary for various reasons, including health, ethical, cultural, or religious beliefs. Understanding and adhering to these restrictions is crucial for overall well-being and respecting individual choices. Here are some common dietary restrictions and considerations:

Religious Dietary Restrictions:

- **Halal:** In Islam, adherents follow specific dietary rules, such as avoiding pork and its by-products, consuming only halal (permissible) meat, and fasting during Ramadan.

- **Kosher:** Observant Jews adhere to kosher dietary laws, which include not mixing dairy and meat, avoiding certain animals, and eating only kosher-certified products.

- **Lent and Fasting:** Many Christian denominations observe periods of fasting and abstinence, particularly during Lent. During these times, specific foods may be restricted.

- **Vegetarianism and Veganism:** Some religious sects or individuals choose to follow vegetarian or vegan diets based on ethical or spiritual beliefs.

Health-Related Dietary Restrictions:

- **Food Allergies:** People with food allergies must avoid specific allergens like nuts, shellfish, gluten, or dairy to prevent allergic reactions.

- **Celiac Disease:** Those with celiac disease must follow a strict gluten-free diet to avoid damaging their small intestine.

- **Diabetes:** People with diabetes often need to monitor their carbohydrate intake, manage their blood sugar levels, and choose low-glycemic foods.

- **High Blood Pressure (Hypertension):** Reducing sodium intake and consuming heart-healthy foods can help manage high blood pressure.

- **Lactose Intolerance:** Individuals with lactose intolerance need to avoid or limit dairy products that contain lactose.

Ethical and Environmental Dietary Choices:

- **Vegetarianism:** Some people choose to abstain from meat for ethical reasons, such as concerns about animal welfare or environmental impact.

- **Veganism:** Vegans avoid all animal products, including dairy and eggs, for similar ethical and environmental concerns.

- **Sustainable Seafood:** Many individuals opt for sustainably sourced seafood to support responsible fishing practices.

Cultural Dietary Preferences:

- **Traditional Diets:** People from different cultural backgrounds often have traditional diets that reflect their heritage and regional cuisine. These diets can be influenced by specific ingredients, cooking methods, and food rituals.

- **Fasting Practices:** Various cultures observe fasting for religious or cultural reasons, such as Ramadan for Muslims and Ekadashi for Hindus.

Weight Management:

- Individuals seeking to gain or lose weight may have dietary restrictions based on their goals and body type. These restrictions can include calorie counting, macronutrient control, and portion management.

2. **Dietary Preferences:**

- Some individuals choose to follow specific diets, such as low-carb, paleo, or Mediterranean diets, based on personal preferences and perceived health benefits.

3. **Allergen Avoidance:** Even if not allergic, some people avoid certain foods like gluten, dairy, or soy for potential health benefits or dietary preferences.

It's important to respect and accommodate these dietary restrictions when cooking for or dining with individuals who have specific needs. When planning meals or eating out, consider these restrictions to ensure everyone's dietary requirements are met. Additionally, it's advisable to consult a healthcare professional or registered dietitian if you have specific dietary concerns or health-related restrictions to ensure you are meeting your nutritional needs while adhering to your dietary choices.

CHAPTER TWO

MEAL PLANNING AND PREP

Creating Balanced Meal Plans

Creating balanced meal plans is essential for maintaining good health and ensuring you get the necessary nutrients your body needs to function properly. A balanced meal typically includes a combination of macronutrients (carbohydrates, proteins, and fats) and micronutrients (vitamins and minerals). Here's a step-by-step guide to creating balanced meal plans:

1. Determine Your Caloric Needs:

- Calculate your daily caloric needs based on factors like age, gender, weight, activity level, and health goals (weight loss, maintenance, or weight gain).

2. Set Macronutrient Ratios:

- Decide on the proportion of macronutrients in your meals. A common approach is to aim for approximately 45-65% of calories from carbohydrates, 10-35% from protein, and 20-35% from fats.

3. Choose Nutrient-Dense Foods:

- Focus on whole, nutrient-dense foods. These are foods rich in vitamins, minerals, fiber, and antioxidants, and they provide more health benefits per calorie consumed.

- Prioritize fruits, vegetables, lean proteins, whole grains, and healthy fats like nuts, seeds, and olive oil.

4. Create a Balanced Plate:

- Use the "plate method" as a visual guide:
    - Fill half your plate with non-starchy vegetables (e.g., leafy greens, broccoli, peppers).
    - Allocate one-quarter of your plate to lean protein sources (e.g., chicken, fish, tofu).
    - Use the remaining quarter for complex carbohydrates or grains (e.g., quinoa, brown rice, sweet potatoes).
    - Include a small serving of healthy fats (e.g., nuts, avocado, olive oil) as well.

5. Plan Your Meals:

- Plan meals that include a variety of food groups. For example:
    - Breakfast: Oatmeal topped with berries and a sprinkle of nuts.
    - Lunch: Grilled chicken with a side of mixed greens and quinoa.
    - Dinner: Baked salmon, steamed broccoli, and brown rice.
    - Snacks: Greek yogurt with honey, or sliced vegetables with hummus.

6. Portion Control:

- Be mindful of portion sizes to avoid overeating. Use measuring tools or visual cues (e.g., a deck of cards for meat) to estimate proper portions.

7. Monitor Sugar and Sodium Intake:

- Minimize added sugars and sodium in your meals. Avoid sugary beverages and processed foods high in added sugars and salt.

8. Include a Variety of Colors:

- A colorful plate often indicates a range of nutrients. Include a variety of fruits and vegetables with different colors for a broad spectrum of vitamins and antioxidants.

9. Hydration:

- Remember to drink plenty of water throughout the day. Avoid excessive sugary or calorie-laden beverages.

10. Meal Timing:

- Eat regular meals and snacks to maintain energy levels and prevent overeating later in the day.

11. Listen to Your Body:

- Pay attention to hunger and fullness cues. Eat when you're hungry and stop when you're satisfied.

12. Seek Professional Guidance:

- If you have specific dietary restrictions, allergies, or medical conditions, consult a registered dietitian or healthcare provider for personalized meal planning.

Balanced meal planning not only supports overall health but also helps with weight management and provides sustained energy throughout the day. Regularly reassess your meal plans and adjust them based on your goals and changing nutritional needs.

SMART SHOPPING FOR HEART AND KIDNEY-FRIENDLY INGREDIENTS

Smart shopping for heart and kidney-friendly ingredients involves selecting foods that are nutritious, low in sodium, and support overall health while considering the dietary restrictions associated with heart and kidney conditions. Here are some tips for smart shopping:

For Heart Health:

Choose Lean Proteins:

- Opt for lean protein sources like skinless poultry, fish (especially fatty fish like salmon and mackerel), lean cuts of beef or pork, and plant-based proteins like beans, lentils, and tofu.

Select Whole Grains:

- Look for whole grains such as brown rice, quinoa, whole wheat pasta, and whole-grain bread. These are high in fiber and can help manage cholesterol levels.

Load Up on Fruits and Vegetables:

- Fill your cart with a variety of colorful fruits and vegetables. They're rich in heart-healthy nutrients and antioxidants. Fresh, frozen, and canned (with no added salt) options are all good choices.

Limit Processed and High-Sodium Foods:

- Avoid or limit highly processed foods, as they often contain excessive sodium, added sugars, and unhealthy fats. Read labels for sodium content and choose lower-sodium options.

Healthy Fats:

- Opt for healthy fats found in sources like avocados, nuts, seeds, and olive oil. These fats can help lower bad cholesterol levels.

Dairy Choices:

- Choose low-fat or fat-free dairy products to reduce saturated fat intake. If you have lactose intolerance, consider lactose-free alternatives.

Snack Smart:

- Select heart-healthy snacks like mixed nuts, Greek yogurt, or fresh fruits. Avoid sugary and salty snacks.

Beverages:

- Stay hydrated with water as your primary beverage. Limit sugary drinks, and consider herbal teas or unsweetened alternatives.

For Kidney Health:

Control Phosphorus and Potassium:

- Kidney patients should monitor their intake of phosphorus and potassium. Avoid high-phosphorus and high-potassium foods like processed meats, dairy products, and high-potassium fruits like bananas and oranges.

Choose Low-Phosphorus Foods:

- Select foods lower in phosphorus, such as fresh vegetables (except for spinach, beet greens, and Swiss chard), rice, pasta, and egg whites.

Limit High-Sodium Foods:

- Kidney patients should watch their sodium intake. Avoid canned soups, processed meats, and salty snacks. Choose lower-sodium or no-salt-added versions of canned goods.

Protein Intake:

- Consult a registered dietitian to determine the appropriate protein intake for your condition. High-quality protein sources like lean meats and fish are often recommended.

Fluid Control:

- If you have fluid restrictions, be mindful of foods with high water content, like watermelon or cucumbers. Measure your fluids carefully, including beverages and foods with a high-water content.

Manage Sugar Levels:

- Kidney patients with diabetes should closely monitor their blood sugar levels and limit sugar intake. Opt for sugar-free or artificially sweetened options when necessary.

Consult a Dietitian:

- Kidney patients, especially those on dialysis, benefit from working with a registered dietitian who can provide personalized dietary guidance and meal planning.

Both for heart and kidney health, reading food labels is crucial to identify hidden sources of sodium, phosphorus, and other nutrients that may be problematic. Remember that smart shopping is the first step in maintaining a heart- and kidney-friendly diet, but proper meal planning and preparation are equally important to ensure you're meeting your nutritional needs while following dietary restrictions.

MEAL PREP TIPS FOR BUSY LIFESTYLES

Meal prepping is a valuable strategy for maintaining a healthy diet, even with a busy lifestyle. It can save time, money, and help you make nutritious choices when you're short on time. Here are some meal prep tips for busy individuals:

1. Plan Your Meals:

- Start by creating a meal plan for the week. Decide which meals you want to prep (breakfast, lunch, dinner, and snacks) and select recipes that are quick and easy to make.

2. Choose Simple Recipes:

- Opt for recipes that are straightforward, require minimal cooking time, and use easily available ingredients. One-pan or one-pot dishes can save both time and clean-up effort.

3. Set a Specific Prep Day:

- Dedicate a specific day of the week for meal prep. Having a routine makes it easier to stick with the practice.

4. Make a Shopping List:

- Create a shopping list based on your meal plan to avoid buying unnecessary items. Stick to your list to save time and money.

5. Batch Cooking:

- Prepare larger batches of meals and portion them into containers for the week. This is particularly useful for dishes that freeze well, such as soups, stews, and casseroles.

6. Invest in Quality Containers:

- Invest in durable, airtight containers to store your prepped meals. Glass containers are a great choice as they are microwave-safe and don't absorb odors.

7. Prepare Ingredients in Advance:

- Wash, chop, and portion vegetables, fruits, and proteins ahead of time. Having ingredients ready to go can significantly speed up meal preparation.

8. Cook in Bulk:

- Make extra portions when cooking dinner, so you have leftovers for lunch the next day. Leftovers can be repurposed into new dishes.

9. Use Frozen Fruits and Vegetables:

- Frozen fruits and vegetables are just as nutritious as fresh ones and can be a convenient addition to your meals. They have a longer shelf life and reduce the need for frequent shopping.

10. Overnight Oats and Chia Pudding:

- Prepare overnight oats or chia pudding the night before, which makes for a quick and nutritious breakfast.

11. Salad Jars:

- Create salad jars with layers of vegetables, protein, and grains. Store the dressing separately until you're ready to eat.

12. Portable Snacks:

- Prepare healthy, portable snacks like mixed nuts, sliced veggies, or fruit that can be easily grabbed on the go.

13. Freeze Extras:

- If you make more than you can consume in a week, freeze extra portions in meal-sized containers for future use.

14. Stay Organized:

- Keep your fridge and pantry well-organized to easily locate prepped meals and ingredients.

15. Be Flexible:

- It's okay to adapt your meal prep based on your schedule. If you can't prepare an entire week's worth of meals, start with a few days and adjust as needed.

16. Try Subscription Meal Kits:

- Subscription meal kit services can provide pre-portioned ingredients and recipes, saving you time on planning and shopping.

17. Remember Food Safety:

- Store prepared meals in the refrigerator within two hours of cooking. Consume them within the recommended timeframes to ensure food safety.

Meal prepping can be a game-changer for busy individuals, helping you stay on track with your health and dietary goals. The key is finding a routine that works for you and simplifying your meal preparation process as much as possible.

CHAPTER THREE

HEART AND KIDNEY-FRIENDLY RECIPES

BREAKFAST

Creating mouth-watering breakfasts that are heart- and kidney-friendly involves selecting ingredients that are low in sodium, phosphorus, and saturated fats while being rich in nutrients like fiber and antioxidants. Here are five delicious recipes, along with ingredients, instructions, and approximate nutritional information:

1. Greek Yogurt Parfait with Berries:

Ingredients:

- 1/2 cup plain Greek yogurt (low-fat or non-fat)
- 1/4 cup fresh or frozen mixed berries (blueberries, strawberries, raspberries)
- 1 tablespoon chopped almonds or walnuts
- 1 teaspoon honey (optional)

Instructions:

1. In a glass or bowl, layer the Greek yogurt.
2. Add the mixed berries on top of the yogurt.
3. Sprinkle the chopped nuts over the berries.
4. Drizzle with honey, if desired.

Nutritional Information:

- Calories: 200-250
- Protein: 14-18g
- Fiber: 3-4g

- Phosphorus: 80-100mg
- Sodium: 40-50mg

2. Quinoa and Vegetable Breakfast Bowl:

Ingredients:

- 1/2 cup cooked quinoa
- 1/4 cup diced cucumber.
- 1/4 cup diced red bell pepper.
- 1/4 cup cherry tomatoes, halved.
- 2 tablespoons fresh parsley, chopped.
- 1 tablespoon lemon juice
- 1 teaspoon olive oil
- Salt-free seasoning to taste

Instructions:

1. In a bowl, combine the cooked quinoa and vegetables.
2. Drizzle with lemon juice and olive oil, and season with salt-free seasoning.
3. Top with chopped parsley.

Nutritional Information:

- Calories: 180-220
- Protein: 5-6g
- Fiber: 4-5g
- Phosphorus: 90-110mg
- Sodium: 5-10mg

3. Spinach and Mushroom Egg White Omelette:

Ingredients:

- 2 egg whites
- 1/4 cup fresh spinach, chopped.
- 1/4 cup mushrooms, sliced.
- 2 tablespoons diced onions.
- 1/2 teaspoon olive oil
- Salt-free seasoning to taste

Instructions:

1. In a non-stick skillet, heat the olive oil over medium heat.
2. Sauté the mushrooms and onions until tender.
3. Add the chopped spinach and cook until wilted.
4. Pour the egg whites over the vegetables, season with salt-free seasoning, and cook until set.

Nutritional Information:

- Calories: 100-120
- Protein: 15-18g
- Fiber: 2-3g
- Phosphorus: 80-100mg
- Sodium: 50-60mg

4. Oatmeal with Apples and Cinnamon:

Ingredients:

- 1/2 cup old-fashioned oats

- 1/2 cup unsweetened applesauce

- 1/2 teaspoon ground cinnamon

- 1 tablespoon chopped almonds or walnuts.

Instructions:

1. Cook the oats according to package instructions.

2. Stir in the unsweetened applesauce and ground cinnamon.

3. Top with chopped nuts.

Nutritional Information:

- Calories: 220-250

- Protein: 5-6g

- Fiber: 5-6g

- Phosphorus: 100-120mg

- Sodium: 0mg

5. Chia Seed Pudding with Mango:

Ingredients:

- 2 tablespoons chia seeds

- 1/2 cup unsweetened almond milk

- 1/4 cup diced mango.

- 1/2 teaspoon vanilla extract

- 1/2 teaspoon honey (optional)

Instructions:

1. In a bowl, mix the chia seeds, almond milk, and vanilla extract.

2. Refrigerate for at least 2 hours or overnight until it thickens.

3. Top with diced mango and drizzle with honey, if desired.

Nutritional Information:

- Calories: 150-180

- Protein: 4-5g

- Fiber: 9-10g

- Phosphorus: 80-100mg

- Sodium: 0mg

These recipes are designed to be heart- and kidney-friendly, but individual dietary needs can vary. It's essential for individuals with kidney conditions to consult a registered dietitian to ensure these recipes are suitable for their specific dietary restrictions and nutritional requirements.

Creating delicious and kidney-friendly lunches that are heart-healthy requires choosing ingredients that are low in sodium, phosphorus, and saturated fats while being rich in nutrients like fiber and antioxidants. Here are five mouth-watering lunch recipes, along with ingredients, instructions, and approximate nutritional information:

1. Quinoa and Black Bean Salad:

Ingredients:

- 1/2 cup cooked quinoa
- 1/2 cup canned low-sodium black beans, drained and rinsed.
- 1/4 cup diced red bell pepper.
- 1/4 cup diced cucumber.
- 2 tablespoons fresh cilantro, chopped.
- 1 tablespoon olive oil
- 1 tablespoon fresh lime juice
- Salt-free seasoning to taste

Instructions:

1. In a bowl, combine the cooked quinoa, black beans, red bell pepper, and cucumber.
2. In a separate bowl, mix the olive oil, lime juice, and salt-free seasoning.
3. Pour the dressing over the salad and toss to combine.
4. Top with chopped cilantro.

- Calories: 300-350
- Protein: 10-12g
- Fiber: 8-10g
- Phosphorus: 120-140mg
- Sodium: 5-10mg

2. Grilled Lemon-Herb Chicken with Steamed Asparagus:

Ingredients:

- 4 ounces boneless, skinless chicken breast
- 1/2 lemon juiced and zested.
- 1/2 teaspoon dried thyme
- 1/2 teaspoon dried rosemary
- 1/2-pound asparagus, trimmed.
- 1 teaspoon olive oil
- Salt-free seasoning to taste

Instructions:

1. Season the chicken with lemon zest, lemon juice, thyme, and rosemary.
2. Grill the chicken until cooked through.
3. Steam the asparagus until tender-crisp.
4. Drizzle the asparagus with olive oil and season with salt-free seasoning.

Nutritional Information:

- Calories: 250-300

- Protein: 30-35g

- Fiber: 4-5g

- Phosphorus: 100-120mg

- Sodium: 10-15mg

3. Baked Salmon with Lemon-Dill Sauce and Sautéed Spinach:

Ingredients:

- 4 ounces salmon fillet

- 1/2 lemon juiced and zested.

- 1 teaspoon fresh dill, chopped.

- 1/2 teaspoon olive oil

- 2 cups fresh spinach

- Salt-free seasoning to taste

Instructions:

1. Season the salmon with lemon zest, lemon juice, and fresh dill.

2. Bake the salmon until cooked through.

3. In a pan, sauté the spinach with olive oil and salt-free seasoning until wilted.

Nutritional Information:

- Calories: 300-350

- Protein: 30-35g

- Fiber: 3-4g

- Phosphorus: 120-140mg

- Sodium: 10-15mg

4. Lentil and Vegetable Soup:

Ingredients:

- 1/2 cup dried green or brown lentils

- 1/2 cup diced carrots.

- 1/2 cup diced celery.

- 1/2 cup diced onions.

- 1 clove garlic, minced.

- 4 cups low-sodium vegetable broth

- 1 teaspoon olive oil

- Salt-free seasoning to taste

Instructions:

1. In a pot, heat the olive oil and sauté the onions and garlic until fragrant.

2. Add the lentils, carrots, and celery, and sauté for a few minutes.

3. Pour in the vegetable broth, bring to a boil, then reduce heat and simmer until the lentils and vegetables are tender.

Nutritional Information:

- Calories: 250-300

- Protein: 15-20g

- Fiber: 12-15g

- Phosphorus: 150-180mg

- Sodium: 40-50mg

5. Mediterranean Chickpea Salad:

Ingredients:

- 1/2 cup canned low-sodium chickpeas, drained and rinsed.

- 1/4 cup diced cucumber.

- 1/4 cup diced tomatoes.

- 2 tablespoons chopped fresh parsley.

- 1 tablespoon olive oil

- 1 tablespoon fresh lemon juice

- Salt-free seasoning to taste

Instructions:

1. In a bowl, combine chickpeas, cucumber, tomatoes, and parsley.

2. In a separate bowl, whisk together the olive oil, lemon juice, and salt-free seasoning.

3. Drizzle the dressing over the salad and toss to combine.

Nutritional Information:

- Calories: 250-300

- Protein: 8-10g

- Fiber: 6-8g

- Phosphorus: 100-120mg

- Sodium: 10-15mg

These recipes are designed to be heart- and kidney-friendly, but individual dietary needs can vary. It's essential for individuals with kidney conditions to consult a registered.

Creating mouth-watering and kidney-friendly dinners for heart health involves selecting ingredients that are low in sodium, phosphorus, and saturated fats while being rich in nutrients like fiber and antioxidants. Here are five delicious dinner recipes, along with ingredients, instructions, and approximate nutritional information:

1. Grilled Lemon Herb Shrimp with Quinoa and Steamed Broccoli:

Ingredients:

- 4 ounces large shrimp, peeled and deveined
- 1/2 lemon, juiced and zested
- 1/2 teaspoon dried oregano
- 1/2 teaspoon dried thyme
- 1/2 cup cooked quinoa
- 1 cup steamed broccoli florets
- 1 teaspoon olive oil
- Salt-free seasoning to taste

Instructions:

1. Season the shrimp with lemon zest, lemon juice, oregano, and thyme.
2. Grill the shrimp until cooked through.
3. Serve over a bed of cooked quinoa and steamed broccoli.
4. Drizzle with olive oil and season with salt-free seasoning.

Nutritional Information:

- Calories: 300-350
- Protein: 30-35g
- Fiber: 5-6g
- Phosphorus: 180-220mg
- Sodium: 10-15mg

2. Baked Chicken Breast with Roasted Vegetables:

Ingredients:

- 4 ounces boneless, skinless chicken breast
- 1 cup mixed vegetables (zucchini, bell peppers, cherry tomatoes)
- 1 teaspoon olive oil
- 1/2 teaspoon dried rosemary
- Salt-free seasoning to taste

Instructions:

1. Season the chicken with dried rosemary and salt-free seasoning.
2. Bake the chicken until cooked through.
3. Toss the mixed vegetables with olive oil and roast until tender.
4. Serve the chicken alongside the roasted vegetables.

Nutritional Information:

- Calories: 250-300

- Protein: 30-35g

- Fiber: 4-5g

- Phosphorus: 160-190mg

- Sodium: 10-15mg

3. Lentil and Vegetable Stir-Fry:

Ingredients:

- 1/2 cup dried green or brown lentils

- 1/2 cup broccoli florets

- 1/2 cup bell peppers, sliced.

- 1/2 cup carrots, sliced.

- 1/4 cup low-sodium stir-fry sauce

- 1 teaspoon olive oil

- Salt-free seasoning to taste

Instructions:

1. Cook the lentils according to package instructions.

2. In a skillet, heat the olive oil and stir-fry the broccoli, bell peppers, and carrots.

3. Add the cooked lentils and stir-fry sauce. Cook until heated through.

4. Season with salt-free seasoning.

Nutritional Information:

- Calories: 300-350

- Protein: 15-20g

- Fiber: 10-12g / Phosphorus: 150-180mg

- Sodium: 60-70mg

4. Baked Cod with Quinoa and Sautéed Spinach:

Ingredients:

- 4 ounces cod fillet
- 1/2 cup cooked quinoa
- 2 cups fresh spinach
- 1 teaspoon olive oil
- 1/2 lemon, juiced and zested
- Salt-free seasoning to taste

Instructions:

1. Season the cod with lemon zest, lemon juice, and salt-free seasoning.
2. Bake the cod until cooked through.
3. In a pan, sauté the spinach with olive oil and salt-free seasoning until wilted.
4. Serve the cod on a bed of cooked quinoa, with sautéed spinach on the side.

Nutritional Information:

- Calories: 300-350
- Protein: 30-35g
- Fiber: 4-5g
- Phosphorus: 180-220mg
- Sodium: 10-15mg

5. Mediterranean Chickpea and Tomato Salad:

Ingredients:

- 1/2 cup canned low-sodium chickpeas, drained and rinsed
- 1/2 cup diced tomatoes
- 1/4 cup diced cucumber
- 2 tablespoons chopped fresh parsley
- 1 tablespoon olive oil
- 1 tablespoon fresh lemon juice
- Salt-free seasoning to taste

Instructions:

1. In a bowl, combine chickpeas, tomatoes, cucumber, and parsley.
2. In a separate bowl, whisk together the olive oil, lemon juice, and salt-free seasoning.
3. Drizzle the dressing over the salad and toss to combine.

Nutritional Information:

- Calories: 250-300
- Protein: 8-10g
- Fiber: 6-8g
- Phosphorus: 100-120mg
- Sodium: 10-15mg

These recipes are designed to be heart- and kidney-friendly, but individual dietary needs can vary. It's essential for individuals with kidney conditions to consult a registered dietitian to ensure these recipes are suitable for their specific dietary restrictions and nutritional requirements.

Creating mouth-watering snacks and desserts that are both heart- and kidney-friendly involves choosing ingredients that are low in sodium, phosphorus, and saturated fats while emphasizing flavors and textures. Here are five delicious snack and dessert recipes, along with ingredients, instructions, and approximate nutritional information:

1. Mixed Berry Parfait:

Ingredients:

- 1/2 cup mixed berries (blueberries, strawberries, raspberries)
- 1/2 cup plain Greek yogurt (low-fat or non-fat)
- 1 tablespoon chopped almonds or walnuts (low phosphorus)
- 1 teaspoon honey (optional)

Instructions:

1. In a glass or bowl, layer half of the mixed berries.
2. Add half of the Greek yogurt.
3. Repeat with the remaining mixed berries and yogurt.
4. Top with chopped nuts and drizzle with honey if desired.

Nutritional Information:

- Calories: 200-250
- Protein: 12-15g

- Fiber: 4-5g

- Phosphorus: 80-100mg

- Sodium: 20-30mg

2. Dark Chocolate-Dipped Strawberries:

Ingredients:

- 4-6 fresh strawberries

- 1 ounce dark chocolate (at least 70% cocoa)

- 1/2 teaspoon coconut oil

- Chopped nuts for topping (optional)

Instructions:

1. Melt the dark chocolate and coconut oil in a microwave or double boiler.

2. Dip each strawberry into the melted chocolate.

3. Place on a parchment paper-lined tray.

4. Sprinkle with chopped nuts if desired.

5. Let cool until the chocolate hardens.

Nutritional Information:

- Calories: 100-150

- Protein: 1-2g

- Fiber: 2-3g

- Phosphorus: 20-30mg

- Sodium: 0-5mg

3. Cinnamon Baked Apples:

Ingredients:

- 1 apple (choose a variety lower in phosphorus, like Gala)
- 1/2 teaspoon cinnamon
- 1 teaspoon honey (optional)
- Chopped nuts for topping (optional)

Instructions:

1. Preheat the oven to 350°F (175°C).
2. Core the apple and slice it into thin rings.
3. Arrange the apple slices on a baking sheet.
4. Sprinkle with cinnamon and drizzle with honey if desired.
5. Bake for 20-25 minutes until the apples are tender.
6. Top with chopped nuts if desired.

Nutritional Information:

- Calories: 100-150
- Protein: 0-1g
- Fiber: 3-4g
- Phosphorus: 10-15mg
- Sodium: 0-5mg

4. Avocado and Tomato Salsa:

Ingredients:

- 1 ripe avocado, diced.
- 1 cup diced tomatoes.
- 1/4 cup diced red onion.
- 1/4 cup fresh cilantro, chopped.
- 1 tablespoon lime juice
- Salt-free seasoning to taste
- Whole-grain crackers for serving.

Instructions:

1. In a bowl, combine the diced avocado, tomatoes, red onion, and cilantro.
2. Drizzle with lime juice and season with salt-free seasoning.
3. Serve the salsa with whole-grain crackers.

Nutritional Information:

- Calories: 150-200
- Protein: 2-3g
- Fiber: 7-8g
- Phosphorus: 50-60mg
- Sodium: 5-10mg

5. Watermelon and Mint Salad:

Ingredients:

- 2 cups cubed watermelon
- 1 tablespoon fresh mint, chopped.
- 1/2 teaspoon lime juice
- 1/2 teaspoon honey (optional)

Instructions:

1. In a bowl, combine the cubed watermelon and chopped mint.
2. Drizzle with lime juice and honey if desired.
3. Toss to combine.

Nutritional Information:

- Calories: 50-70
- Protein: 1g
- Fiber: 1-2g
- Phosphorus: 10-15mg
- Sodium: 0-5mg

These snacks and desserts are designed to be heart- and kidney-friendly, but individual dietary needs can vary. It's essential for individuals with kidney conditions to consult a registered dietitian to ensure these recipes are suitable for their specific dietary restrictions and nutritional requirements.

Creating delicious beverages that are both heart- and kidney-friendly involves choosing ingredients that are low in sodium, phosphorus, and saturated fats while providing a refreshing and tasty experience. Here are five mouth-watering beverage recipes, along with ingredients, instructions, and approximate nutritional information:

1. Watermelon Cooler:

Ingredients:

- 2 cups cubed and seedless watermelon.
- 1/2 lime, juiced.
- A few fresh mint leaves.
- Ice cubes

Instructions:

1. Blend the watermelon until smooth.
2. Add lime juice and fresh mint leaves, and blend again.
3. Pour over ice and garnish with additional mint leaves if desired.

Nutritional Information:

- Calories: 60-80
- Protein: 1-2g
- Fiber: 1-2g
- Phosphorus: 10-20mg
- Sodium: 0mg

2. Berry Blast Smoothie:

Ingredients:

- 1/2 cup mixed berries (blueberries, strawberries, raspberries)
- 1/2 cup low-fat or non-fat plain Greek yogurt
- 1/2 banana
- 1/2 cup unsweetened almond milk
- Ice cubes (optional)

Instructions:

1. Combine all the ingredients in a blender.
2. Blend until smooth and creamy.
3. Add ice cubes if you want a colder smoothie.

Nutritional Information:

- Calories: 150-200
- Protein: 10-12g
- Fiber: 4-5g
- Phosphorus: 120-140mg
- Sodium: 50-60mg

3. Cucumber and Mint Infused Water:

Ingredients:

- 6-8 slices of cucumber
- A few sprigs of fresh mint
- 1 quart of water
- Ice cubes

Instructions:

1. Place the cucumber slices and fresh mint in a pitcher.
2. Add water and let it sit in the refrigerator for a few hours or overnight.
3. Serve chilled over ice.

Nutritional Information:

- Calories: 0
- Protein: 0g
- Fiber: 0g
- Phosphorus: 0mg
- Sodium: 0mg

4. Hibiscus Iced Tea:

Ingredients:

- 2 hibiscus tea bags
- 4 cups boiling water
- 2-3 tablespoons honey (optional)
- Lemon slices and mint leaves for garnish (optional)

Instructions:

1. Place the hibiscus tea bags in a heatproof pitcher.
2. Pour boiling water over the tea bags and let steep for about 5 minutes.
3. Remove the tea bags and stir in honey if desired.
4. Let it cool to room temperature, then refrigerate until cold.

5. Serve with lemon slices and mint leaves if desired.

Nutritional Information:

- Calories: 0 (without honey), 60-80 (with honey)
- Protein: 0g
- Fiber: 0g
- Phosphorus: 0mg
- Sodium: 0mg

5. Green Tea and Mango Smoothie:

Ingredients:

- 1 green tea bag
- 1/2 cup hot water
- 1/2 cup diced mango (choose low-phosphorus variety)
- 1/2 banana
- 1/2 cup low-fat or non-fat plain Greek yogurt
- Ice cubes (optional)

Instructions:

1. Brew the green tea in hot water and let it cool.
2. In a blender, combine the brewed green tea, diced mango, banana, and Greek yogurt.
3. Blend until smooth.
4. Add ice cubes if you want a colder smoothie.

Nutritional Information:

- Calories: 150-200
- Protein: 10-12g

- Fiber: 2-3g

- Phosphorus: 70-90mg

- Sodium: 40-50mg

These beverages are designed to be heart- and kidney-friendly, but individual dietary needs can vary. It's essential for individuals with kidney conditions to consult a registered dietitian to ensure these recipes are suitable for their specific dietary restrictions and nutritional requirements.

CHAPTER FOUR

RECIPES BY DISEASE STAGE

Early-Stage Heart and Kidney Disease

In the early stages of heart and kidney disease, it's crucial to focus on a heart- and kidney-friendly diet that's low in sodium, saturated fats, and phosphorus, while being rich in nutrients like fiber and antioxidants. Here are some recipes suitable for early-stage heart and kidney disease:

1. Early-Stage Heart and Kidney-Friendly

Breakfast: Quinoa and Berries Breakfast Bowl

Ingredients:

- 1/2 cup cooked quinoa
- 1/4 cup mixed berries (blueberries, strawberries, raspberries)
- 2 tablespoons chopped almonds (low phosphorus)
- 1/2 teaspoon honey (optional)

Instructions:

1. In a bowl, layer the cooked quinoa.
2. Add the mixed berries on top.
3. Sprinkle with chopped almonds and drizzle with honey if desired.

2. Early-Stage Heart and Kidney-Friendly Lunch: Mediterranean Chickpea Salad

Ingredients:

- 1/2 cup canned low-sodium chickpeas, drained and rinsed
- 1/4 cup diced cucumber
- 1/4 cup diced tomatoes
- 2 tablespoons chopped fresh parsley
- 1 tablespoon olive oil
- 1 tablespoon fresh lemon juice
- Salt-free seasoning to taste

Instructions:

1. In a bowl, combine the chickpeas, cucumber, tomatoes, and parsley.
2. Drizzle with olive oil and lemon juice.
3. Season with salt-free seasoning.

3. Early-Stage Heart and Kidney-Friendly Dinner: Baked Salmon with Lemon-Dill Sauce and Steamed Asparagus

Ingredients:

- 4 ounces salmon fillet
- 1/2 lemon, juiced and zested
- 1 teaspoon fresh dill, chopped
- 1/2 pound asparagus, trimmed

- 1 teaspoon olive oil

- Salt-free seasoning to taste

Instructions:

1. Season the salmon with lemon zest, lemon juice, and fresh dill.

2. Bake the salmon until cooked through.

3. Steam the asparagus until tender-crisp.

4. Drizzle the asparagus with olive oil and season with salt-free seasoning.

4. Early-Stage Heart and Kidney-Friendly Snack:

Mixed Berry Parfait

Ingredients:

- 1/2 cup plain Greek yogurt (low-fat or non-fat)

- 1/4 cup mixed berries (blueberries, strawberries, raspberries)

- 1 tablespoon chopped almonds (low phosphorus)

- 1 teaspoon honey (optional)

Instructions:

1. In a glass or bowl, layer the Greek yogurt.

2. Add the mixed berries on top of the yogurt.

3. Sprinkle with chopped almonds and drizzle with honey if desired.

5. Early-Stage Heart and Kidney-Friendly Dessert: Cinnamon Baked Apples

Ingredients:

- 1 apple (choose a variety lower in phosphorus, like Gala)
- 1/2 teaspoon cinnamon
- 1 teaspoon honey (optional)
- Chopped nuts for topping (optional)

Instructions:

1. Preheat the oven to 350°F (175°C).
2. Core the apple and slice it into thin rings.
3. Arrange the apple slices on a baking sheet.
4. Sprinkle with cinnamon and drizzle with honey if desired.
5. Bake for 20-25 minutes until the apples are tender.
6. Top with chopped nuts if desired.

These recipes are suitable for individuals in the early stages of heart and kidney disease, but it's essential to consult a healthcare provider or a registered dietitian to tailor the diet to your specific condition and dietary requirements.

MODERATE STAGE HEART AND KIDNEY DISEASE

In the moderate stages of heart and kidney disease, it's crucial to follow a heart- and kidney-friendly diet that remains low in sodium, saturated fats, and phosphorus. Additionally, you may need to limit certain nutrients, such as potassium and protein. Here are some recipes suitable for individuals in the moderate stages of heart and kidney disease:

1. Moderate-Stage Heart and Kidney-Friendly Breakfast: Oatmeal with Banana and Almonds

Ingredients:

- 1/2 cup old-fashioned oats
- 1/2 banana, sliced (choose a ripe banana for lower potassium)
- 1 tablespoon chopped almonds (low phosphorus)
- 1/2 teaspoon cinnamon
- 1 teaspoon honey (optional)

Instructions:

1. Cook the oats according to package instructions.
2. Top with sliced banana, chopped almonds, and a sprinkle of cinnamon.
3. Drizzle with honey if desired.

2. Moderate-Stage Heart and Kidney-Friendly Lunch: Quinoa and Roasted Vegetable Salad

Ingredients:

- 1/2 cup cooked quinoa
- 1 cup roasted vegetables (zucchini, bell peppers, cherry tomatoes)
- 1 tablespoon olive oil
- 1/2 lemon, juiced and zested
- Salt-free seasoning to taste

Instructions:

1. Combine the cooked quinoa and roasted vegetables in a bowl.
2. Drizzle with olive oil and lemon juice.
3. Season with salt-free seasoning.

3. Moderate-Stage Heart and Kidney-Friendly Dinner: Baked Cod with Lemon-Dill Sauce and Sautéed Spinach

Ingredients:

- 4 ounces cod fillet
- 1/2 cup cooked quinoa
- 2 cups fresh spinach
- 1 teaspoon olive oil
- 1/2 lemon, juiced and zested.
- Salt-free seasoning to taste

Instructions:

1. Season the cod with lemon zest, lemon juice, and salt-free seasoning.

2. Bake the cod until cooked through.

3. In a pan, sauté the spinach with olive oil and salt-free seasoning until wilted.

4. Serve the cod on a bed of cooked quinoa, with sautéed spinach on the side.

4. Moderate-Stage Heart and Kidney-Friendly Snack: Cucumber and Mint Tzatziki

Ingredients:

- 1/2 cucumber, finely grated and drained
- 1/2 cup low-fat or non-fat Greek yogurt
- 1 clove garlic, minced.
- 1 tablespoon fresh mint, chopped.
- Salt-free seasoning to taste
- Whole-grain crackers or low-sodium pita for dipping

Instructions:

1. Mix the grated cucumber, Greek yogurt, minced garlic, and fresh mint.

2. Season with salt-free seasoning.

3. Serve with whole-grain crackers or low-sodium pita.

5. Moderate-Stage Heart and Kidney-Friendly Dessert: Baked Apple Slices with Cinnamon and Yogurt

Ingredients:

- 1 apple (choose a variety lower in phosphorus, like Gala)
- 1/2 teaspoon cinnamon
- 1/2 cup low-fat or non-fat Greek yogurt
- 1 teaspoon honey (optional)

Instructions:

1. Preheat the oven to 350°F (175°C).
2. Core the apple and slice it into thin rings.
3. Arrange the apple slices on a baking sheet.
4. Sprinkle with cinnamon.
5. Bake for 15-20 minutes until the apples are tender.
6. Serve with a dollop of Greek yogurt and drizzle with honey if desired.

These recipes are suitable for individuals in the moderate stages of heart and kidney disease. However, it's essential to consult a healthcare provider or a registered dietitian to tailor the diet to your specific condition and dietary requirements.

ADVANCED STAGE HEART AND KIDNEY DISEASE

In the advanced stages of heart and kidney disease, dietary restrictions become more stringent, and it's crucial to limit sodium, phosphorus, potassium, and fluids. Here are some recipes suitable for individuals in the advanced stages of heart and kidney disease:

1. Advanced-Stage Heart and Kidney-Friendly Breakfast: Egg White Omelette with Spinach and Toast

Ingredients:

- 3 egg whites
- 1/4 cup fresh spinach, chopped
- 1/2 teaspoon olive oil
- 1 slice low-sodium whole-grain bread

Instructions:

1. In a non-stick skillet, heat the olive oil over medium heat.
2. Sauté the chopped spinach until wilted.
3. Pour the egg whites over the spinach and cook until set.
4. Serve with a toasted slice of low-sodium whole-grain bread.

2. Advanced-Stage Heart and Kidney-Friendly Lunch: Low-Potassium Vegetable Soup

Ingredients:

- 1/2 cup diced zucchini.
- 1/2 cup diced yellow squash.
- 1/4 cup diced carrots.
- 1/4 cup diced celery.
- 1/4 cup diced onions.
- 1 clove garlic, minced.
- 4 cups low-sodium vegetable broth
- 1 teaspoon olive oil
- Salt-free seasoning to taste

Instructions:

1. In a pot, heat the olive oil and sauté the onions and garlic until fragrant.
2. Add the diced zucchini, yellow squash, carrots, and celery and sauté for a few minutes.
3. Pour in the low-sodium vegetable broth, bring to a boil, then reduce heat and simmer until the vegetables are tender.
4. Season with salt-free seasoning.

3. Advanced-Stage Heart and Kidney-Friendly Dinner: Baked Tilapia with Mashed Cauliflower

Ingredients:

- 4 ounces tilapia fillet
- 1/2 head of cauliflower, chopped.
- 1/2 teaspoon olive oil
- 1/2 lemon, juiced and zested.
- Salt-free seasoning to taste

Instructions:

1. Season the tilapia with lemon zest and salt-free seasoning.
2. Bake the tilapia until cooked through.
3. Steam the chopped cauliflower until tender, then mash with a potato masher or a food processor.
4. Drizzle with olive oil, lemon juice, and season with salt-free seasoning.

4. Advanced-Stage Heart and Kidney-Friendly Snack: Rice Cake with Hummus

Ingredients:

- 1 rice cake (low-sodium)
- 2 tablespoons low-potassium hummus

Instructions:

1. Spread the low-potassium hummus over the rice cake.
2. Enjoy as a kidney-friendly snack.

5. Advanced-Stage Heart and Kidney-Friendly Dessert: Baked Pear with Cinnamon

Ingredients:

- 1 ripe pear (choose a variety lower in potassium)
- 1/2 teaspoon cinnamon

Instructions:

1. Preheat the oven to 350°F (175°C).
2. Slice the pear in half and remove the core.
3. Sprinkle each half with cinnamon.
4. Bake for 20-25 minutes until the pear is tender.

These recipes are designed to meet the dietary restrictions of individuals in the advanced stages of heart and kidney disease, but it's crucial to consult a healthcare provider or a registered dietitian for personalized guidance and to ensure these recipes align with your specific condition and nutritional needs.

DIALYSIS-FRIENDLY RECIPES

For individuals on dialysis, it's essential to follow a strict dietary regimen that includes limited sodium, phosphorus, and potassium intake. Here are some dialysis-friendly recipes tailored to meet these specific dietary requirements:

1. Dialysis-Friendly Breakfast: Egg White and Vegetable Scramble

Ingredients:

- 3 egg whites
- 1/4 cup diced red bell pepper.
- 1/4 cup diced zucchini.
- 1/4 cup diced onions.
- 1/4 cup diced mushrooms.
- 1/2 teaspoon olive oil
- Salt-free seasoning to taste

Instructions:

1. In a non-stick skillet, heat the olive oil over medium heat.
2. Sauté the onions and mushrooms until soft.
3. Add the red bell pepper and zucchini and cook until tender.
4. Pour in the egg whites and cook until set.
5. Season with salt-free seasoning.

2. Dialysis-Friendly Lunch: Low-Potassium Chicken Salad

Ingredients:

- 3 ounces cooked, skinless chicken breast, diced.
- 1/4 cup diced cucumber.
- 1/4 cup diced celery.
- 1/4 cup diced carrots.
- 1 tablespoon low-potassium mayonnaise
- Salt-free seasoning to taste

Instructions:

1. In a bowl, combine the diced chicken, cucumber, celery, and carrots.
2. Mix in the low-potassium mayonnaise.
3. Season with salt-free seasoning.

3. Dialysis-Friendly Dinner: Poached Salmon with Steamed Asparagus

Ingredients:

- 4 ounces poached salmon fillet
- 1/2 pound asparagus, trimmed
- 1/2 lemon, juiced and zested
- Salt-free seasoning to taste

Instructions:

1. Poach the salmon in simmering water until it flakes easily with a fork.

2. Steam the asparagus until tender-crisp.

3. Drizzle with lemon juice and zest.

4. Season with salt-free seasoning.

4. Dialysis-Friendly Snack: Rice Cake with Low-Potassium Almond Butter

Ingredients:

- 1 rice cake (low-sodium)
- 1-2 tablespoons low-potassium almond butter

Instructions:

1. Spread the low-potassium almond butter over the rice cake.

2. Enjoy this low-potassium snack.

5. Dialysis-Friendly Dessert: Baked Apple Slices with Cinnamon

Ingredients:

- 1 apple (choose a variety lower in potassium)
- 1/2 teaspoon cinnamon

Instructions:

1. Preheat the oven to 350°F (175°C).

2. Core the apple and slice it into thin rings.

3. Arrange the apple slices on a baking sheet.

4. Sprinkle with cinnamon.

5. Bake for 15-20 minutes until the apples are tender.

These dialysis-friendly recipes are tailored to meet the dietary restrictions of individuals undergoing dialysis treatment. However, it's crucial to consult a healthcare provider or a registered dietitian for personalized guidance and to ensure these recipes align with your specific condition and nutritional needs.

CHAPTER FIVE

INGREDIENT SUBSTITUTIONS

Tips for Substituting Ingredients

Substituting ingredients in recipes can be a useful strategy for adapting to dietary restrictions or specific health conditions. Here are some tips for substituting ingredients at various disease stages:

1. Lower-Sodium Substitutes:

- **Herbs and Spices:** Use herbs and spices like rosemary, thyme, basil, and oregano to add flavor instead of salt.

- **Low-Sodium Broth:** Substitute low-sodium or homemade broth for regular broth in recipes.

2. Lower-Fat Substitutes:

- **Greek Yogurt:** Use Greek yogurt instead of sour cream or mayonnaise in dips and dressings to reduce saturated fat.

- **Applesauce or Mashed Bananas:** Replace butter or oil with unsweetened applesauce or mashed bananas in baking recipes.

3. Lower-Sugar Substitutes:

- **Stevia or Erythritol:** Use sugar substitutes like stevia or erythritol in place of sugar for sweetening beverages and desserts.

- **Fresh Fruit:** Sweeten dishes naturally with fresh fruits like mashed bananas, dates, or pureed prunes.

4. Lower-Phosphorus Substitutes (for Kidney Disease):

- **Rice Milk or Almond Milk:** Substitute dairy milk with rice milk or almond milk, which typically have lower phosphorus content.

- **Fresh Vegetables:** Opt for fresh vegetables over canned ones to reduce phosphorus intake.

5. Lower-Potassium Substitutes (for Kidney Disease):

- **Lower-Potassium Fruits:** Choose lower-potassium fruits like apples, berries, and grapes instead of high-potassium options.

- **Cauliflower:** Replace high-potassium potatoes with cauliflower in mashed dishes.

6. Lower-Protein Substitutes (for Kidney Disease):

- **Tofu:** Substitute tofu for meat or poultry in recipes to reduce protein content.

- **Egg Whites:** Use egg whites instead of whole eggs to reduce protein in dishes.

7. Lower-Fluid Substitutes (for Kidney Disease):

- **Gelatin-Based Desserts:** Make gelatin-based desserts for a treat that's lower in fluids compared to traditional puddings or ice cream.

- **Thicker Sauces:** Thicken sauces with cornstarch or potato starch instead of using excess liquid.

8. Gluten-Free Substitutes (for Celiac Disease):

- **Gluten-Free Flour Blends:** Replace wheat flour with gluten-free flour blends in recipes to create gluten-free baked goods.

- **Rice or Corn Pasta:** Use rice or corn pasta instead of wheat pasta in pasta dishes.

When making substitutions, it's important to consider the specific dietary needs and restrictions of the individual. Consultation with a registered dietitian or healthcare provider is advisable for guidance tailored to a particular health condition or dietary requirement. Additionally, keep in mind that the taste and texture of the dish may vary with substitutions, so it might take some experimentation to achieve the desired results.

LOW-SODIUM ALTERNATIVES

Reducing sodium intake is essential for those with heart and kidney disease or high blood pressure. Here are some low-sodium alternatives to common high-sodium ingredients:

1. Herbs and Spices:

- Use herbs like rosemary, thyme, basil, oregano, and parsley to season your dishes.

- Experiment with spices such as garlic powder, onion powder, paprika, cumin, and turmeric for flavor.

2. Low-Sodium Broth:

- Opt for low-sodium or no-salt-added broths when making soups, stews, and sauces.

- Consider making homemade broth without added salt.

3. Fresh Citrus:

- Replace salt with fresh lemon or lime juice to enhance the taste of your meals.

4. Vinegar:

- Use vinegar, such as balsamic, apple cider, or red wine vinegar, to add tanginess and flavor to salads and dishes.

5. Low-Sodium Soy Sauce or Tamari:

- Choose low-sodium soy sauce or tamari for a reduced-sodium alternative in Asian-inspired recipes.

6. Low-Sodium Canned Vegetables:

- Look for canned vegetables labeled "low-sodium" or "no salt added" as a convenient alternative.

7. Unsalted Butter or Margarine:

- Use unsalted butter or margarine in recipes that call for butter to control sodium intake.

8. Salt-Free Seasoning Blends:

- Explore salt-free seasoning blends that are readily available in stores or make your own by mixing various herbs and spices.

9. Low-Sodium Condiments:

- Choose condiments like low-sodium ketchup, low-sodium mustard, and low-sodium mayonnaise when needed.

10. Fresh Garlic and Onions:

- Use fresh garlic and onions to infuse dishes with flavor without relying on salt.

11. Low-Sodium Salsa:

- Incorporate low-sodium salsa into Mexican and Tex-Mex recipes for extra flavor.

12. Nutritional Yeast:

- Nutritional yeast can provide a savory, cheese-like flavor to dishes without added sodium.

13. Roasted or Grilled Vegetables:

- Roasting or grilling vegetables intensifies their natural flavors without needing added salt.

14. No-Salt-Added Canned Beans:

- Select canned beans labeled "no salt added" for a sodium-conscious choice.

15. Low-Sodium Broth-Based Sauces:

- Use low-sodium, broth-based sauces for stir-fries and other dishes.

Remember to read food labels carefully to identify hidden sources of sodium, and gradually reduce your salt intake to allow your taste buds to adjust to lower sodium levels. Over time, you'll become accustomed to enjoying the natural flavors of foods without excessive salt.

For individuals with kidney disease, managing potassium and phosphorus intake is essential. Here are some modifications and alternatives to help control these minerals in your diet:

1. Potassium Modifications:

- **Choose Low-Potassium Fruits:** Opt for lower-potassium fruits like apples, berries, grapes, and pears instead of high-potassium options like bananas, oranges, and dried fruits.

- **Reduce Tomato Products:** Limit your intake of tomatoes and tomato-based products, as they are high in potassium.

- **Soak Potatoes:** If you enjoy potatoes, peel and soak them in water for several hours before cooking to reduce their potassium content.

- **Limit Avocado:** Avocado is high in potassium, so consume it in moderation or choose low-potassium alternatives.

- **Use Rice Milk or Almond Milk:** Substitute dairy milk with rice milk or almond milk, which typically have lower potassium content.

- **Boil or Soak High-Potassium Vegetables:** High-potassium vegetables like potatoes, sweet potatoes, and spinach can have their potassium reduced by boiling or soaking in water.

2. Phosphorus Modifications:

- **Choose Low-Phosphorus Proteins:** Select lean cuts of meat, poultry, and fish as they typically contain less phosphorus than organ meats.

- **Limit Dairy Products:** Restrict your intake of dairy products, especially hard cheeses, which are high in phosphorus.

- **Use Egg Whites:** Instead of whole eggs, use egg whites in recipes to reduce phosphorus intake.

- **Low-Phosphorus Grains:** Opt for low-phosphorus grains such as white rice, white bread, and pasta instead of whole grains.

- **Avoid Colas and Dark Sodas:** Dark sodas often contain phosphoric acid, which can increase phosphorus levels. Opt for clear sodas or water.

- **Phosphate Binders:** Some individuals may require phosphate binders to help control phosphorus absorption. Consult with your healthcare provider about their use.

Remember to work closely with a registered dietitian or healthcare provider to create a dietary plan tailored to your specific needs. They can help you manage potassium and phosphorus while ensuring you still receive the necessary nutrients for overall health. Additionally, routine monitoring of your blood levels for these minerals is crucial to assess how well you are managing your dietary modifications.

CHAPTER SIX

QUICK AND EASY SOLUTIONS

15-Minute Heart and Kidney-Friendly Meals

Creating quick, heart- and kidney-friendly meals is possible with some simple and nutritious recipes. Here are a few 15-minute meal ideas that fit these criteria:

1. Grilled Lemon Herb Chicken:

- Marinate boneless, skinless chicken breast in lemon juice, olive oil, and herbs.

- Grill for about 6-7 minutes per side.

- Serve with a side of steamed green beans and quinoa.

2. Seared Salmon with Dill Sauce:

- Sear salmon fillets in a non-stick skillet for about 4-5 minutes per side.

- Prepare a dill sauce by mixing low-fat Greek yogurt, fresh dill, and lemon juice.

- Serve the salmon with the dill sauce and a side of asparagus or broccoli.

3. Shrimp Stir-Fry:

- Sauté shrimp, colorful bell peppers, and snap peas in a stir-fry sauce made with low-sodium soy sauce, ginger, and garlic.

- Serve over brown rice or cauliflower rice.

4. Mediterranean Chickpea Salad:

- Combine canned chickpeas, cherry tomatoes, cucumber, olives, and feta cheese.
- Drizzle with olive oil and balsamic vinegar and sprinkle with fresh basil.
- Serve with whole-grain pita bread.

5. Spinach and Mushroom Omelette:

- Whisk eggs or egg whites with a pinch of salt-free seasoning.
- Sauté sliced mushrooms and spinach until wilted.
- Pour the egg mixture over the veggies and cook until set, folding it in half.

6. Tuna Salad Bowl:

- Mix canned tuna with low-sodium mayonnaise, diced celery, and pickles.
- Serve over a bed of fresh greens and cherry tomatoes.

7. Quick Quinoa and Vegetable Bowl:

- Cook quinoa according to package instructions.
- Top with sautéed or steamed low-potassium vegetables and a sprinkle of your favorite herbs.

8. Caprese Salad Wrap:

- Fill a whole grain wrap with fresh mozzarella, tomato slices, basil leaves, and a drizzle of balsamic reduction.

9. Mediterranean Hummus and Veggie Wrap:

- Spread hummus on a whole-grain wrap.

- Add sliced cucumbers, bell peppers, cherry tomatoes, and black olives.

- Roll it up and enjoy.

10. Simple Lentil Soup: Heat low-sodium vegetable or chicken broth and canned lentils in a pot. - Add chopped spinach or kale and season with salt-free seasoning.

These meals are quick, heart- and kidney-friendly options that provide essential nutrients and flavors. Always adjust recipes to meet your specific dietary needs and consult with a healthcare provider or registered dietitian for guidance on portion control and ingredient choices.

ONE-POT RECIPES FOR SIMPLICITY

One-pot recipes are not only simple but also convenient for those with heart and kidney health concerns. Here are some one-pot recipes that are easy to prepare and considerate of dietary restrictions:

1. One-Pot Vegetable and Rice Pilaf:

- In a large pot, sauté diced onions and garlic in olive oil until fragrant.

- Add rice and cook for a few minutes, stirring to coat with oil.

- Stir in low-sodium vegetable broth, diced carrots, bell peppers, and peas.

- Season with salt-free seasoning, cover, and simmer until the rice is tender and the liquid is absorbed.

2. One-Pot Chicken and Quinoa Casserole:

- In a large oven-safe pot, brown boneless, skinless chicken thighs.

- Add quinoa, low-sodium chicken broth, and a mix of vegetables like broccoli and bell peppers.

- Season with herbs and spices.

- Cover and bake in the oven until the chicken is cooked, and the quinoa is tender.

3. One-Pot Lentil and Spinach Soup:

- In a large pot, sauté onions and garlic in olive oil until softened.

- Add dried green or brown lentils, low-sodium vegetable broth, diced tomatoes, and a generous handful of spinach.

- Simmer until the lentils are tender.

4. One-Pot Mediterranean Pasta:

- In a large skillet, combine whole-grain pasta, canned low-sodium chickpeas, cherry tomatoes, olives, and diced red onions.

- Add low-sodium vegetable broth, olive oil, and Mediterranean herbs.

- Cook until the pasta is done, and the sauce has thickened.

5. One-Pot Turkey and Vegetable Stir-Fry:

- In a large skillet, brown lean ground turkey with garlic and ginger.

- Add a mix of stir-fry vegetables like broccoli, snap peas, and bell peppers.

- Stir in a low-sodium stir-fry sauce and serve over brown rice.

6. One-Pot Spinach and Artichoke Orzo:

- In a large pot, sauté chopped onions and garlic in olive oil.

- Stir in orzo pasta, low-sodium vegetable broth, canned artichoke hearts, and fresh spinach.

- Cook until the pasta is tender and the mixture is creamy.

7. One-Pot Chili:

- In a large pot, brown lean ground turkey or beef.

- Add kidney beans, black beans, diced tomatoes, chili powder, cumin, and other seasonings.

- Simmer until flavors meld, and the chili thickens.

These one-pot recipes offer simplicity, easy preparation, and considerate ingredients for heart and kidney health. Remember to adjust seasonings and ingredients based on your specific dietary needs and consult with a healthcare provider or registered dietitian for personalized guidance.

Seasonal Ingredient Guides

Eating seasonally can be an excellent way to incorporate fresh and local ingredients into your heart and kidney-friendly diet. Here are seasonal ingredient guides for spring, summer, fall, and winter:

Spring Season:

- **Fruits:** Strawberries, cherries, apricots, and rhubarb.
- **Vegetables:** Asparagus, spinach, peas, artichokes, and spring greens.
- **Herbs:** Fresh basil, mint, and chives.
- **Protein:** Light fish such as tilapia, and skinless poultry.
- **Grains:** Barley and bulgur.
- **Dairy:** Low-fat yogurt and cheese.

Summer Season:

- **Fruits:** Berries (blueberries, raspberries, strawberries), watermelon, peaches, and plums.
- **Vegetables:** Zucchini, tomatoes, bell peppers, eggplant, and corn.
- **Herbs:** Fresh cilantro, dill, and parsley.
- **Protein:** Grilled chicken and lean cuts of beef.
- **Grains:** Quinoa and whole-grain couscous.
- **Dairy:** Low-fat milk and yogurt.

Fall Season:

- **Fruits:** Apples, pears, grapes, and cranberries.
- **Vegetables:** Pumpkins, sweet potatoes, Brussels sprouts, and butternut squash.
- **Herbs:** Rosemary, sage, and thyme.
- **Protein:** Turkey and lean cuts of pork.
- **Grains:** Brown rice and whole wheat pasta.
- **Dairy:** Low-fat or non-fat dairy products.

Winter Season:

- **Fruits:** Citrus fruits (oranges, grapefruits), kiwi, and pomegranates.
- **Vegetables:** Brussels sprouts, kale, cabbage, and carrots.
- **Herbs:** Cilantro and chives.
- **Protein:** Salmon, tofu, and lean cuts of beef.
- **Grains:** Oats and barley.
- **Dairy:** Low-fat or non-fat dairy products.

Incorporating seasonal ingredients into your meals can enhance the flavor of your dishes and provide a variety of nutrients. Seasonal foods are often fresher and more affordable, making it easier to create heart and kidney-friendly recipes. Don't forget to adapt recipes and portion sizes to suit your specific dietary needs and consult with a healthcare provider or registered dietitian for personalized guidance.

Creating seasonal menus is a wonderful way to enjoy fresh, flavorful, and heart- and kidney-friendly meals throughout the year. Here are sample seasonal menus for each season:

Spring Menu:

Appetizer:

- **Asparagus Soup:** A creamy, low-sodium soup made with fresh asparagus.

Main Course:

- **Grilled Lemon Herb Chicken:** Marinated in lemon juice, olive oil, and fresh herbs.
- **Quinoa Salad:** With fresh peas, cherry tomatoes, and a light vinaigrette.

Side Dish:

- **Steamed Artichokes:** Served with a lemony dip.

Dessert:

- **Strawberry Parfait:** Layer fresh strawberries, low-fat yogurt, and a sprinkle of granola.

Summer Menu:

Appetizer:

- **Caprese Salad:** Sliced tomatoes, fresh mozzarella, basil, and a balsamic reduction.

Main Course:

- **Grilled Salmon:** With a zesty lemon-dill sauce.

- **Cucumber and Tomato Salad:** Dressed with olive oil and fresh herbs.

Side Dish:

- **Grilled Corn on the Cob:** Lightly brushed with olive oil.

Dessert:

- **Watermelon and Mint Salad:** A refreshing and hydrating treat.

Fall Menu:

Appetizer:

- **Butternut Squash Soup:** Creamy and spiced with nutmeg and cinnamon.

Main Course:

- **Herb-Roasted Turkey Breast:** Served with a cranberry and orange relish.

- **Mashed Sweet Potatoes:** Seasoned with a touch of cinnamon and low-sodium butter.

- **Roasted Brussels Sprouts:** Tossed with olive oil and balsamic glaze.

Dessert:

- **Baked Pears:** Sprinkled with cinnamon and served with low-fat Greek yogurt.

Winter Menu:

Appetizer:

- **Roasted Beet and Citrus Salad:** A colorful and flavorful salad.

Main Course:

- **Baked Cod with Lemon-Dill Sauce:** A light and heart-healthy fish dish.

- **Quinoa Pilaf:** With roasted winter vegetables.

- **Garlic and Lemon Broccoli:** A simple, healthy side.

Dessert:

- **Mixed Berry Compote:** Warm mixed berries topped with a dollop of low-fat Greek yogurt.

These seasonal menus emphasize fresh, in-season ingredients while keeping heart and kidney health in mind. Adapt and modify recipes as needed based on specific dietary requirements and consult with a healthcare provider or registered dietitian for personalized guidance.

CHAPTER EIGHT

COOKING TECHNIQUES

Reducing Sodium in Cooking

Reducing sodium in cooking is essential for heart and kidney health. Here are some strategies and tips to help you cut down on sodium while still enjoying flavorful meals:

1. Use Fresh Herbs and Spices:

- Season your dishes with fresh herbs like basil, thyme, rosemary, and spices like garlic, ginger, and cumin to enhance flavor without relying on salt.

2. Create Homemade Seasoning Blends:

- Make your own salt-free seasoning blends by mixing herbs, spices, and aromatics. Experiment with different combinations until you find your favorite flavor profiles.

3. Limit Salt in Recipes:

- Gradually reduce the amount of salt you add to recipes. You may find that you need less salt than the recipe calls for.

4. Choose Low-Sodium Broths and Canned Goods:

- Opt for low-sodium or no-salt-added broths, canned vegetables, and beans when possible.

5. Rinse Canned Vegetables:

- If you use canned vegetables, rinse them under running water to remove some of the excess sodium.

6. Use Fresh Produce:

- Choose fresh fruits and vegetables over canned or processed ones whenever you can.

7. Read Food Labels:

- Pay attention to food labels and select products with lower sodium content. Look for items labeled "low-sodium" or "no salt added."

8. Cook from Scratch:

- Preparing meals from scratch allows you to have complete control over the ingredients, including salt.

9. Marinate Meats and Poultry:

- Marinating meat and poultry in flavorful, low-sodium mixtures can infuse them with taste.

10. Choose Low-Sodium Condiments:

Use low-sodium soy sauce, low-sodium tomato paste, and other condiments that have reduced salt content.

11. Fresh Citrus Juice: Enhance the taste of your dishes with fresh lemon or lime juice.

12. Taste Before You Add: Taste your food before adding any salt to ensure it genuinely needs more seasoning.

13. Cook with Non-Stick Cookware: Non-stick cookware requires less oil, which can reduce the need for salt in some dishes.

14. Limit Processed Foods: Processed foods often contain high levels of sodium, so minimize their consumption.

15. Gradual Adjustment: Reducing sodium is a gradual process. Your taste buds will adapt over time, and you'll become more sensitive to the natural flavors of food.

By implementing these strategies, you can significantly reduce sodium in your cooking while still enjoying tasty and heart- and kidney-friendly meals. Remember that a gradual reduction in salt is more likely to be sustainable and allow your palate to adjust to lower sodium levels.

PHOSPHORUS MANAGEMENT IN RECIPES

Phosphorus management is essential for individuals with kidney disease, as high phosphorus levels can contribute to health complications. Here are some tips for managing phosphorus in recipes:

1. Choose Low-Phosphorus Proteins:

- Opt for low-phosphorus protein sources, such as chicken, turkey, fish, and egg whites, over high-phosphorus options like organ meats and processed meats.

2. Limit Dairy and Dairy Substitutes:

- Dairy products are typically high in phosphorus. Choose low-phosphorus or phosphorus-free alternatives like almond milk or rice milk.

3. Use Phosphorus Binders:

- If prescribed by your healthcare provider, take phosphorus binders with meals to reduce phosphorus absorption.

4. Avoid High-Phosphorus Additives:

- Watch out for additives like phosphate salts (e.g., disodium phosphate) in processed foods and read labels carefully.

5. Modify Whole Grains:

- Whole grains like brown rice are higher in phosphorus than refined grains. You can reduce phosphorus by soaking or rinsing grains before cooking.

6. Choose Low-Phosphorus Vegetables:

- Include low-phosphorus vegetables like green beans, cabbage, and cauliflower in your recipes. Limit high-phosphorus ones like spinach and potatoes.

7. Be Cautious with Nuts and Seeds:

- Nuts and seeds can be high in phosphorus. Consume them in moderation and consider soaking them to reduce phosphorus content.

8. Make Low-Phosphorus Sauces:

- When preparing sauces and gravies, use low-phosphorus broths and thickeners like cornstarch instead of high-phosphorus ingredients.

9. Reduce Phosphorus in Baking:

- In baking, substitute buttermilk with a mixture of milk and vinegar or lemon juice to reduce phosphorus content.

10. Limit High-Phosphorus Condiments: - Be cautious with high-phosphorus condiments like Worcestershire sauce, soy sauce, and certain hot sauces.

11. Watch Portions: - Pay attention to portion sizes and maintain appropriate portion control, as even low-phosphorus foods can contribute to phosphorus intake when consumed excessively.

It's essential to consult with a registered dietitian or healthcare provider to develop a personalized meal plan that aligns with your specific dietary needs and restrictions. They can provide guidance on managing phosphorus while maintaining a balanced and nutritious diet.

COOKING METHODS FOR HEALTHIER MEALS

Using healthier cooking methods can help you prepare heart and kidney-friendly meals. Here are some cooking methods that focus on minimizing unhealthy fats and sodium while retaining flavor and nutrition:

1. Grilling:

- Grilling allows excess fat to drip away from food, making it a heart-healthy option.

- For extra flavor, marinate lean meats, poultry, or fish in herbs, spices, and low-sodium marinades.

2. Baking or Roasting:

- Baking and roasting are great ways to cook proteins and vegetables without adding excessive fats.

- Season with herbs, spices, and a small amount of heart-healthy oils.

3. Steaming:

- Steaming is an excellent way to preserve the nutrients in vegetables while requiring no added fats.

- Steam vegetables like broccoli, carrots, and green beans for a kidney-friendly side dish.

4. Sautéing or Stir-Frying:

- Use a small amount of heart-healthy oil (e.g., olive oil) to sauté or stir-fry ingredients.

- Include plenty of fresh vegetables and lean proteins.

5. Poaching:

- Poaching is a gentle cooking method that can be used for fish and chicken.

- Use a flavorful broth for poaching, and add fresh herbs and spices for taste.

6. Griddling or Pan-Searing:

- When griddling or pan-searing, use a non-stick pan to minimize the need for excess fats.

- Lightly oil the pan or use cooking spray.

7. Slow Cooking:

- Slow cookers are ideal for making heart-healthy soups and stews.

- Use lean cuts of meat and add plenty of vegetables and herbs for flavor.

8. Microwaving:

- Microwaving is a quick and convenient way to cook vegetables and grains with minimal added fats and sodium.

- Use microwave-safe containers with a lid to trap steam and preserve nutrients.

9. Use Non-Stick Cookware:

- Non-stick pans and pots require less oil for cooking and are easier to clean.

10. Healthy Dressings and Sauces: - Prepare homemade dressings and sauces with heart-healthy oils, vinegar, and herbs instead of high-fat, high-sodium store-bought options.

11. Seasoning with Herbs and Spices: - Replace salt with herbs and spices to add flavor to your dishes without extra sodium.

12. Low-Sodium Broths and Stocks: - Use low-sodium or homemade broths and stocks as a base for soups and stews to control sodium intake.

Incorporating these cooking methods into your meal preparation can help you create healthier, heart and kidney-friendly dishes that are still full of flavor. Additionally, consulting with a registered dietitian or healthcare provider can provide personalized guidance on your specific dietary needs.

Here's the nutrient breakdown for each of the recipes provided:

1. Grilled Lemon Herb Chicken with Quinoa Pilaf and Asparagus:

- **Grilled Lemon Herb Chicken (per serving):**
    - Calories: Approximately 150-200 calories
    - Protein: 25-30 grams
    - Fat: 3-5 grams
    - Carbohydrates: 0 grams (assuming no marinade)
    - Fiber: 0 grams
    - Sodium: Minimal, depending on the marinade used
- **Quinoa Pilaf (per serving):**
    - Calories: Approximately 150-200 calories
    - Protein: 5-8 grams
    - Fat: 3-5 grams
    - Carbohydrates: 25-30 grams
    - Fiber: 2-3 grams
    - Sodium: Minimal, depending on the broth used
- **Asparagus (per serving):**
    - Calories: Approximately 20-40 calories

- Protein: 2-4 grams

- Fat: 0-1 gram

- Carbohydrates: 4-8 grams

- Fiber: 2-4 grams

- Sodium: Minimal, especially if lightly seasoned

2. Seared Salmon with Dill Sauce and Quinoa and Grilled Vegetable Salad:

- **Seared Salmon (per serving):**

  - Calories: Approximately 200-250 calories

  - Protein: 20-25 grams

  - Fat: 10-15 grams (heart-healthy fats)

  - Carbohydrates: 0 grams

  - Fiber: 0 grams

  - Sodium: Minimal, depending on the seasoning

- **Dill Sauce (per serving):**

  - Calories: Approximately 20-30 calories

  - Protein: 1-2 grams

  - Fat: 1-2 grams (heart-healthy fats)

  - Carbohydrates: 2-3 grams

  - Fiber: 0 grams

  - Sodium: Minimal, depending on the recipe

- **Quinoa and Grilled Vegetable Salad (per serving):**

- Calories: Approximately 150-200 calories

- Protein: 4-6 grams

- Fat: 5-8 grams (heart-healthy fats)

- Carbohydrates: 25-30 grams

- Fiber: 4-6 grams

- Sodium: Minimal, depending on the seasoning and dressing

These nutrient breakdowns are approximate and can vary based on specific ingredients and preparation methods. Be sure to adjust recipes to your dietary requirements, especially if you have specific health concerns. For precise nutrient information, consult with a registered dietitian who can tailor your meal plan to your specific needs.

Here are the details for dietary fiber, protein, sodium, potassium, and phosphorus in each of the recipes provided:

1. Grilled Lemon Herb Chicken with Quinoa Pilaf and Asparagus:

- **Dietary Fiber:**
    - Grilled Lemon Herb Chicken: Minimal
    - Quinoa Pilaf: 2-3 grams per serving
    - Asparagus: 2-4 grams per serving

- **Protein:**
    - Grilled Lemon Herb Chicken: 25-30 grams per serving
    - Quinoa Pilaf: 5-8 grams per serving
    - Asparagus: 2-4 grams per serving

- **Sodium:**
    - The sodium content varies depending on the marinade and seasoning used. Be cautious with sodium if you have dietary restrictions.

- **Potassium:**
    - Grilled Lemon Herb Chicken: Approximately 200-250 mg per serving
    - Quinoa Pilaf: Approximately 100-150 mg per serving

- Asparagus: Approximately 200-300 mg per serving

- **Phosphorus:**

  - Grilled Lemon Herb Chicken: Minimal phosphorus

  - Quinoa Pilaf: Minimal phosphorus

  - Asparagus: Minimal phosphorus

2. Seared Salmon with Dill Sauce and Quinoa and Grilled Vegetable Salad:

- **Dietary Fiber:**

  - Seared Salmon: Minimal

  - Dill Sauce: Minimal

  - Quinoa and Grilled Vegetable Salad: 4-6 grams per serving

- **Protein:**

  - Seared Salmon: 20-25 grams per serving

  - Dill Sauce: 1-2 grams per serving

  - Quinoa and Grilled Vegetable Salad: 4-6 grams per serving

- **Sodium:**

  - The sodium content varies depending on the seasoning and dressing used. Be cautious with sodium if you have dietary restrictions.

- **Potassium:**

  - Seared Salmon: Approximately 300-350 mg per serving

- Dill Sauce: Approximately 40-60 mg per serving

- Quinoa and Grilled Vegetable Salad: Approximately 200-250 mg per serving

- **Phosphorus:**

  - Seared Salmon: Approximately 200-250 mg per serving

  - Dill Sauce: Minimal phosphorus

  - Quinoa and Grilled Vegetable Salad: Approximately 100-150 mg per serving

These details provide a general overview of the nutrient content in each recipe. Actual nutrient values can vary based on specific ingredients, portion sizes, and preparation methods. For precise nutrient information tailored to your dietary needs, consult with a registered dietitian or use nutrition analysis tools to calculate the exact values based on the ingredients you use.

CHAPTER TEN

FAMILY-FRIENDLY OPTIONS

Recipes The Whole Family Will Love

Creating heart and kidney-friendly recipes that the whole family can enjoy is both delicious and nutritious. Here are some family-friendly recipes:

1. Baked Chicken Tenders with Sweet Potato Fries:

- **Ingredients:**
    - Chicken tenders (use skinless, boneless chicken breast)
    - Sweet potatoes, cut into fries
    - Olive oil
    - Whole-grain breadcrumbs
    - Garlic powder, paprika, and Italian seasoning for seasoning
    - Low-sodium ketchup or a yogurt-based dip
- **Instructions:**
1. Preheat the oven to 425°F (220°C).

2. Toss sweet potato fries in olive oil, season with a pinch of salt-free seasoning, and bake until crispy.

3. Dip chicken tenders in olive oil, then coat with whole-grain breadcrumbs and seasoning.

4. Place the chicken tenders on a baking sheet and bake until cooked through.

5.   Serve with sweet potato fries and a side of low-sodium ketchup or a yogurt-based dip.

2. Vegetable and Black Bean Quesadillas:

- **Ingredients:**
    - Whole-grain tortillas
    - Black beans (canned, low-sodium)
    - Bell peppers, onions, and zucchini (sliced)
    - Low-fat cheese
    - Salsa (low-sodium)
- **Instructions:**

1.   Sauté sliced vegetables in a non-stick skillet until tender.

2.   Lay a tortilla flat and layer it with black beans, sautéed vegetables, and a sprinkle of low-fat cheese.

3.   Place another tortilla on top.

4.   Heat the quesadilla in the skillet until the cheese melts and the tortillas are golden.

5.   Serve with salsa.

3. Turkey and Veggie Meatballs with Whole-Grain Pasta:

- **Ingredients:**
    - Lean ground turkey
    - Grated zucchini and carrot
    - Whole-grain pasta
    - Low-sodium tomato sauce

- Garlic, oregano, and basil for seasoning

- **Instructions:**

1. Mix lean ground turkey with grated zucchini and carrot, and season with garlic, oregano, and basil.

2. Form the mixture into meatballs and bake until cooked through.

3. Cook whole-grain pasta and heat low-sodium tomato sauce.

4. Serve the meatballs over the pasta with the tomato sauce.

4. Veggie-Packed Stir-Fry:

- **Ingredients:**

    - Lean protein (chicken, tofu, or shrimp)

    - Assorted vegetables (bell peppers, broccoli, snap peas, carrots)

    - Low-sodium stir-fry sauce

    - Brown rice or quinoa

- **Instructions:**

1. Stir-fry lean protein and vegetables in a non-stick skillet with a minimal amount of oil.

2. Add low-sodium stir-fry sauce and serve over brown rice or quinoa.

These recipes are heart and kidney-friendly and can be enjoyed by the whole family. Feel free to customize them to suit your family's taste preferences and consult with a registered dietitian for personalized guidance based on specific dietary needs.

Getting Kids Involved in Healthy Cooking

Getting kids involved in healthy cooking is a fantastic way to teach them about nutrition, instill good eating habits, and create enjoyable family experiences. Here are some tips on how to involve kids in the kitchen:

1. Age-Appropriate Tasks:

- Assign tasks that are suitable for their age and skill level. Younger children can wash vegetables, stir ingredients, or set the table, while older kids can help with more complex tasks.

2. Plan Together:

- Let kids participate in meal planning. Discuss what meals to prepare, consider their preferences, and make a shopping list together.

3. Choose Kid-Friendly Recipes:

- Start with simple, kid-friendly recipes that are easy to prepare and appeal to their tastes. For example, homemade whole-wheat pizza, fruit smoothies, or colorful salads.

4. Teach Basic Skills:

- Show them how to safely use kitchen tools like knives (depending on their age), graters, and measuring cups. Teach them about proper hand-washing and hygiene.

5. Explore Ingredients:

- Take the opportunity to educate kids about different ingredients, their nutritional value, and where they come from.

6. Get Creative:

- Encourage creativity in the kitchen. Let them experiment with flavors and presentation.

7. Hands-On Cooking:

- Allow kids to actively participate in every step, from washing and cutting to mixing and cooking.

8. Encourage Healthy Choices:

- Explain the importance of choosing healthy ingredients, like whole grains, lean proteins, and lots of colorful vegetables.

9. Be Patient:

- Be patient with their learning process and the inevitable mess that comes with it. Remember, it's a learning experience.

10. Make it Fun: - Cooking should be enjoyable. Play music, have a dance party, or create a game related to the cooking process.

11. Praise and Positive Reinforcement: - Offer praise for their efforts and let them know how much you appreciate their help in the kitchen.

12. Share Meals Together: - After cooking, sit down together as a family to enjoy the meal. Discuss the flavors and what they liked about it.

13. Teach Food Safety: - Explain the importance of food safety, such as proper food storage, avoiding cross-contamination, and cooking meat to a safe temperature.

14. Gradual Independence: - Over time, give them more independence in the kitchen. They can eventually prepare simple meals on their own with your supervision.

Involving kids in healthy cooking not only teaches them valuable life skills but also helps create a positive attitude towards nutritious foods. It's an excellent way to bond as a family and share the joy of preparing and enjoying meals together.

CONCLUSION

In conclusion, heart and kidney health is of paramount importance for maintaining overall well-being. By understanding the common causes and symptoms of heart and kidney diseases, you can take proactive steps to prevent and manage these conditions. Nutrition plays a vital role in disease management, making it crucial to focus on key nutrients, portion control, and dietary restrictions.

Creating balanced meal plans, smart shopping for heart and kidney-friendly ingredients, and efficient meal prep can simplify the process of maintaining a heart and kidney-friendly diet. Moreover, it's essential to tailor your approach to different disease stages, including early-stage, moderate-stage, advanced-stage, and dialysis-friendly recipes.

When making dietary choices, consider factors like reducing sodium, managing potassium and phosphorus, and ensuring an adequate intake of dietary fiber and protein. Utilizing healthy cooking methods and involving kids in cooking can make the journey to heart and kidney health an enjoyable and educational experience for the whole family.

Remember that consulting with a healthcare provider or registered dietitian is crucial for creating a personalized plan that meets your specific needs and restrictions. By prioritizing heart and kidney health through informed choices and a well-balanced diet, you can take significant steps toward a healthier and more fulfilling life.